HEALTHY WORK

Putting the Good Back Into Work

SCOTT GODWIN, MS

Foreword by Marion Glover
President, Glover Capital, Inc.

Roots Publishing®

Healthy Work

*"Man, the subject, is the purpose of work,
not the objects it brings about."*
-RJ Snell

Contents

Contents

Foreword for *Healthy Work*

As someone who at 73 is asked almost daily by friends *"When are you going to stop working?"* my answer is *"I don't know"*. I honestly don't know because my wife (who works with me) and I rarely think about it, since our work is such an enjoyable part of our life. Working and contributing is part of who we are and what we're all about.

Scott Godwin's book *Healthy Work* identifies how all people of all backgrounds and education levels, even in the latter stage of their life, can find work a healthy and rewarding endeavor. We feel so rewarded when we help a client work through a complex, difficult situation and when we see a project through to the end. It provides my wife and me a meaningful purpose. There is an irreplaceable feeling of satisfaction in getting the job done right and doing the best we can every time.

Yes, work can most certainly be both healthy and fun at the same time and it's a joyful thing when approached the right way. This superb book will show you how to get there in your own working life.

I couldn't recommend more to study this book carefully and re-read it again and again, using it as a lifetime guide to find *Healthy Work* in your life.

Marion Glover, CFP
Glover Capital

About Marion Glover

Prior to founding Glover Capital, Mr. Glover worked for more than fourteen years for The Coca-Cola Company, where he attained the positions of Vice President of Corporate Strategic Planning and Vice President of Corporate Financial Planning and Information Systems. Mr. Glover has also served as President of Edwards Baking Company and President of Peterson Companies. He has a Securities Principal license and is a Dean's list graduate of Georgia Tech where he is a trustee emeritus of the Georgia Tech Foundation, earned an M.B.A. from Harvard Business School and was the recipient of a J. Spencer Love Fellowship.

1

—

Introduction: *Work is good.*

"What Ranks Above All Else for Economic and Political Reconstruction Is a Radical Change of Ideologies. Economic Prosperity Is Not So Much a Material Problem; It Is, First of All, an Intellectual, Spiritual, and Moral Problem."   *– Ludwig Von Mises*

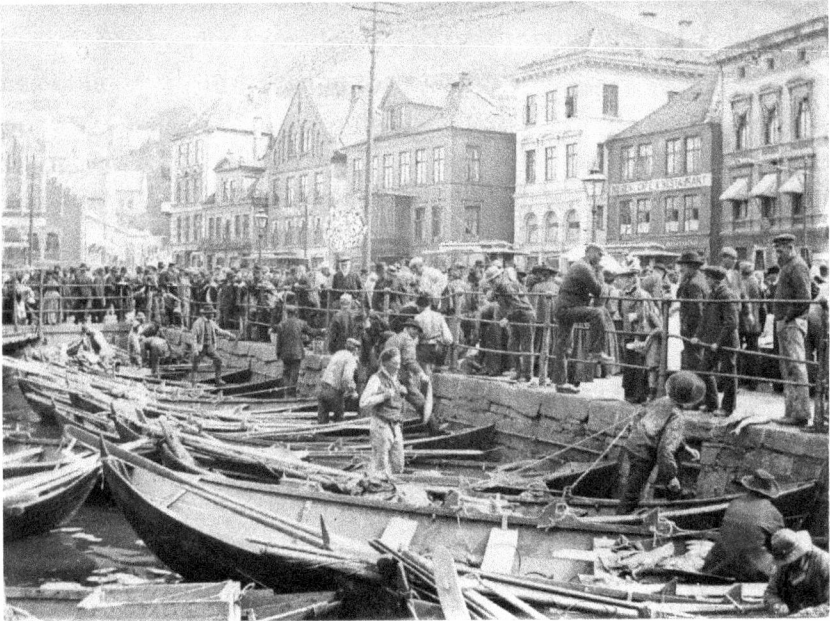

Fish Market, 1890

We as Americans will spend much of our lives working. Sometimes we work so much that we don't stop to think about why we work and what our work means to us. Working really is a way of life. Work is a choice. Work is a philosophy. We choose to work, or we choose not to. Work is a crucial part of who we are as individuals and as a nation. It doesn't matter what type of work we do or how much money we make, if we view our own lives as important, then our work will be important. Whether it's mentally, physically, or spiritually, how we approach our work will also have a huge impact on our health. We should take work seriously.

Based on the enthusiastic feedback I got in regard to my first book, *Movement & Meaning* (about the effect of exercise on mental health) and the sections in it which emphasized the importance of a healthy working life, I decided to tackle the topic of work and what exactly makes it healthy, thus the title of this book- *Healthy Work*. Look at this book first and foremost as a defense of the nobility and pure goodness of work, from the simplest of tasks to the most complex engineering, technology, medicine, or finance. This book is coming along at the right time: the American Middle Class is now a quickly shrinking minority.(1) It's getting harder as workers in America so it's a good time to take a step back and take a critical look at work and what it means and how we can make it as healthy of an endeavor as possible.

Work is a good thing and in this book, I want to bring joy to your working life. It sounds simple, but for work to be healthy we must first say that work is good. Unfortunately, it has become difficult to say that work is a good thing because the values we live with in modern America are confusing. We aren't all living by the same script. Americans have many different value systems. We don't all believe the same things. It's hard to say what exactly is "good" and so it's hard as a result to say, "work is good" in and of itself. This is not a positive development because without being able to take pride in the simple goodness of work, we're robbing ourselves of a great source of joy, happiness, and health.

The illustrated figure is a mythical *Ouroboros*, a snake swallowing its own tail, which represents self-destruction. A dilemma we face in the modern world is that of a value-less and nihilistic society. A society which values nothing could eventually destroy itself like the *Ouroboros* because it will have nothing left to

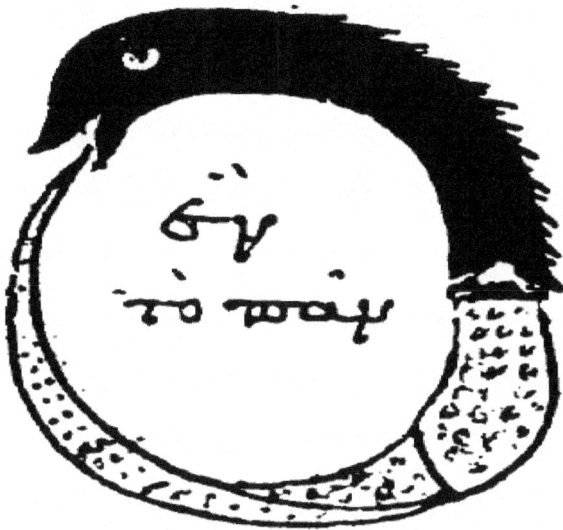

uphold as good- no basis in reality, no meaning, and nothing to declare or to defend or fight for as "good" or "bad", including work. If we can't say anything is good for certain, how can we say that work is good?

But work is good. Rational behavior, grounded in reality and morality, requires judgement and discriminate thought. For us to say something is good we must first say "good" exists in the first place. We must judge work to be good and to discriminately prefer work over non-work, for it to have a positive meaning. *Equality* and *tolerance* are the dominant values in modern America. These two values are indeed important as part of a larger framework of values, but when it comes to work we must be willing to go further than equality and tolerance and say that work is without a doubt good in its own right. Equality and tolerance are not enough to uphold work as good. Here's why:

As common sense as it sounds to say that "work is good", if a modern liberal society like ours values only equality and tolerance then we must tolerate non-work, or slothfulness, or non-contribution as an equal "good." To make work healthy and meaningful we must move beyond equality and tolerance to a more inclusive and comprehensive view of what constitutes a "good" way of life. We must ensure equal protection and opportunity, but not equal outcomes. We must also tolerate behaviors and people we find difficult to deal with, and those whom we disagree with, so long as they aren't doing things which are illegal and they don't endanger others.

If, on the other hand, absolute equality and tolerance are all we have left to value, then to say this is "good" or this is "bad" we will always be in violation of our values and not be able to say that work is one way or the other, good or bad. For to tolerate everything is to endorse anarchy, and to ensure equal outcome is to render life meaningless- and so *Ouroboros* swallows its tail, and at the end of the Super Bowl no one wins. For the game to make sense, whether it's chess, football, or life, we need to agree on what the rules are.

All the same, when we say, "people should work", or "it's good to work" we are making a value judgement which bumps up against the ideology of non-judgmental thinking and its core values of equality and tolerance. This is not politics, this is true. Sadly, it's become polarizing and even controversial in some circles to simply say "work is good".

Because if we say, "people should work" we are saying that men or women who don't work or won't work and who are a purposeful drain on society should not be treated as equals to working men and women, nor should this behavior be looked at as good to any degree. We must, in other words, treat working people and people who refuse to contribute as existing on differing planes of moral existence. JFK famously asked, *"ask not what your country can do for you, but what you can do for your country."* This is the essence of healthy work, asking "what can I do to contribute?", because contribution is a good thing.

In order for work to be deemed good and meaningful, we must rationally judge the opposite to not be. Without bad, there is no such thing as good, and vice versa. In order to judge or to discriminately choose between two or more options, we must think and be rational.

We must decide how to act, think, and judge in our own best interests but also in the best interests of the community and world in which we live. When it comes to work, we must ask, what is best in life? No matter your political viewpoint, there's no doubt that the value of work has been degraded as the overall values of America have declined. American icon Booker T. Washington once said *"Nothing ever comes to one, that is worth having, except as a result of hard work."* Work is a good thing, a noble thing, and a virtuous thing.

When I ponder work and what it means to me I think about many things. I think about the essence of man's existence, the purpose of a man's life, and what is abhorrent and repulsive and what is virtuous and noble. I think of the satisfaction of being mentally and physically tired at the end of a work day. I consider the satisfaction of looking in the mirror and saying to myself: "I did the best I could. My work is done, for today." I consider the gnawing guilt I feel when I know I could have done better. Most of all, when I think of work, I think of values.

The "good" is also the *why* of work. The "good" is the motivation, because the good spurs the movement and effort of work, and the meaning. Good climbs in the house to put out the fire, risking life and limb. Good brings the volunteers out to a Special Olympics event. Good takes a bullet for a comrade. Good spurs the teacher to be a little more patient with the student. Good forms the civic clubs, the hospitals, the businesses, and the charities.

Many in our culture, including me at times, have forgotten the inherent wisdom, beauty, and rejuvenating power of core human virtues and values such as *commitment, loyalty, respect, service, love, self-restraint, courage, discipline, compassion, bravery,* and *honesty,* among others. Without these core values, there is nothing- no meaning, no joy, and no goodness. Many in our age have experienced and have taken valueless and self-destructive paths in life. I know because I've met them, counseled them, and struggled with them.

As changing as the world may be, it is built upon something. In order for anything to become, *it must first be.* A good healthy working life is built on values. Values are built upon revealed truths and wisdom of the past about what is best in life. Some things in this world truly are better than others. Values allowed civilization to be built and sustained and will always be important. Values created man and allowed him to evolve and become more self-aware. Men made valuable alliances, they were loyal, virtuous, and cooperative and so they adapted and survived.

Some political agendas portray capitalism as bad, and it most certainly has a downside when corrupted. Capitalism and the technologies of finance aside though, trade is itself one of the single greatest forces for peace, flourishing, stability, survival, and technological progress the world has ever known. Work, craftsmanship, and the specialization of labor are defining characteristics of mankind. Men valued the right things and so they worked, cooperated, traded, progressed, survived, and thrived.

CS Lewis, in his classic book "Abolition of Man" writes of a future valueless time when men may no longer be men at all- *men without chests* he calls them. Like the branches of a tree attacking the roots, man as we know him may not survive if he gets too far from the roots, or values, of his existence, if he forgets the lessons learned from the past about what is good. Without values, man can destroy himself. Too often, when work is not valued, I'm afraid that's what happens. Work is a wonderfully good thing but when we don't value it like we should, it loses its meaning and vitality.

One of the more memorable experiences I've had in my life occurred while traveling in Moscow, Russia in the Underground Subway Train Stations in 2013. As part of the communist propaganda machine, the Soviet dictator Josef Stalin sponsored the creation in the 1930s what came to be known as surrealist art, which considerably dramatizes the heroic virtues of the Russian proletariat (working class) and rural agricultural society in statues and paintings lining the walls of the Underground. This artwork, priceless amounts of which can still be found in the Moscow underground, is breathtakingly beautiful despite Stalin's flawed totalitarian Marxist philosophy.

Seeing this art made an unforgettable impression upon me. The Russian surrealist art is meant to elevate the consciousness of the common worker as he passes through the underground, and make him feel part of an epic ideological struggle for workers' justice. Again, despite the evil and totalitarian nature of the Soviet regime, this particular art really is beautiful and so is the concept- work is beautiful and good, and we should know this to be true every day of our working life.

Though work is itself noble and good, the working man or woman, the wage-earner, the hourly worker, in America has not seen his or her wages rise (adjusted for inflation) since the 1970s. Globalization has not been good for many American workers. Even many college graduates are finding themselves unemployed or underemployed, with thousands of dollars of debt. Men in particular are highly sensitive to status, much more than women, and modern work challenges have undoubtedly had a negative influence on the American working man's psyche and mental health, as well as on his role within society and within the family. Evidence is plentiful: crime, divorce, depression, alcoholism, drug abuse, and a lack of committed parenting is prevalent in a growing number of working class families. This demise of a healthy working life is even more clearly evident in the now virtually non-existent, nuclear black family.

At the very least, as we struggle through the challenges of a rapidly changing world, we should do everything we can to celebrate the simple goodness of work at every opportunity. We should celebrate and uphold all types of work, from all types of people. If men want to do work more traditionally viewed as work for women, so be it. If women want to be executives, or police officers, or have a large family and stay home, more power to them.

The point is that work and contribution are healthy things and should be celebrated as innately good. Work, if it is to be a healthy endeavor, requires us to make judgements. We must say that we were made to work, trade, and cooperate, to contribute. Work is part of who we are. We are born to work and to produce, not just consume. Whether the community banker, the forklift driver, the math teacher, the plumber, the IT Specialist, or the office janitor we must recognize the uncompromising and inherent moral goodness of all work. For work to be healthy, it must be meaningful, and meaning comes from values. The worker should be proud of his chosen way of life because work it is a good thing.

Work is a way of life. It is a way of being, a rational, intellectual, spiritual, and moral choice, and a way of seeing the world and our place in it. We choose to work and create value, and thus do good, or we choose not to.

healthy work

2

What is the Purpose of Work?
To Create Value & Fulfill Human
Needs & Desires

"Try not to become a man of success, but rather try to become a man of value." —Albert Einstein

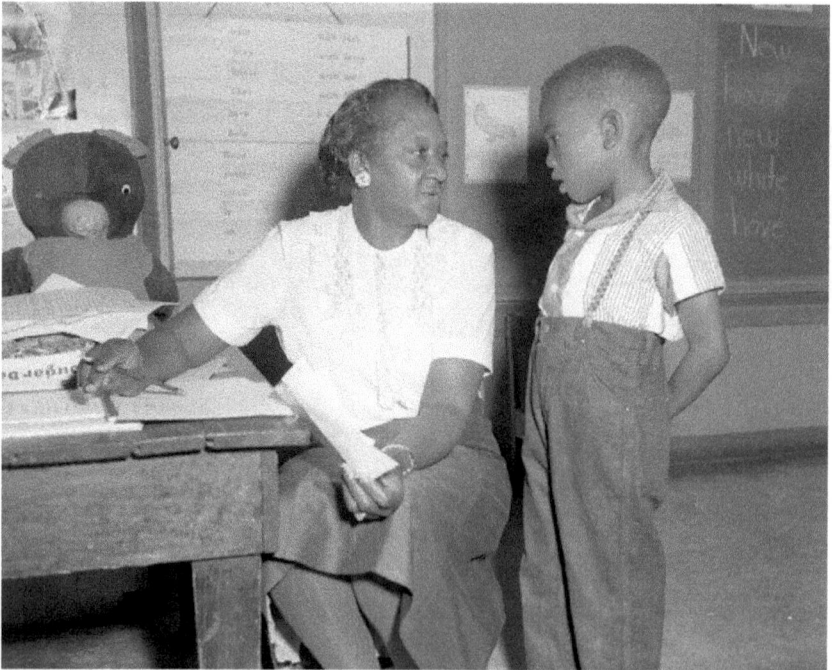

Teacher & Student, 1957

healthy work

Men and women work for many different reasons because individuals have different desires and goals. Some men, like Donald Trump or Barrack Obama, work politically to become powerful because they enjoy the intoxication of power or because they feel a duty to steer the nation into a direction they see as best. Some people work simply to put food on the table and to keep a roof over their head. Others work to travel, so that they make enough money to have adventurous lives. A good parent works to raise their children to be healthy adults. We can't say what exactly people should work for, because individuals value economic goods, services, and other things differently.

Some value free time above all, so they work only enough time to acquire the basic means of survival, so they can use their free time in leisure or hobbies. Others may have a goal to acquire $10,000,000 in their lifetime. Some people work because they enjoy working. It is not usually up to us to judge whether why someone works or what they work for is "right / good" or "wrong / bad". Value judgements about how much, how hard, and how long someone works are largely subjective, because every person is different in how they value the fruits of their labor, in their views about their own life and its purpose, and in how they view the world around them.

As we covered in the introduction, if we want work to be healthy we must say work is a good thing. Otherwise, work would have no real meaning. The purpose of all reasonable work, work which itself is noble and is done for various reasons, is regardless always done to create value, for business owners, entrepreneurs, capitalists, and workers themselves, and to fulfill the human needs and desires of each, no matter how different they might be.

In some parts of the world, rural India or Mexico for example, low-income workers work so they will have enough money to buy groceries or to pay a utility bill. On the far other side of the economic spectrum, highly educated young professional New Yorkers might be working to create value in order that they can make enough money to retire at 40. In all cases, the worker works to create value in the marketplace so to fulfill his or her desires. This sounds like common sense because it is, but it's worth repeating-work is done to create value.

Capitalists, savers, entrepreneurs, and employers are driven to create value in different capacities. In the case of the *capitalist*, the goal is to create financial value through lending and earned interest and in the case of the *entrepreneur*, the goal is to create something the market values so that the person might acquire value through money or other goods. The *saver* has an excess of value and stores it, usually in the form of gold or money, and hopes to use it more efficiently later. The *employee* creates value in his work and earns a wage or salary, then does what he can or must with it.

Since the purpose of work is to create value, work which is not valuable has no rational purpose or meaning and should not be done, unless one wants to act irrationally (which people do). It sounds obvious, but it's worth pointing out: to do meaningless work which creates no value is a waste of time. Even worse than wasting time, work which is destroying net value or is illegal is destructive to all parties involved. If someone partakes to steal or destroy through his labor, he is actually taking value away both from himself on a moral and spiritual level and from society on an economic basis, aside from the fact that he may end up in jail. Work should always be done to create value, not take value away. Work that does not create value in some form is at its best futile, unreasonable, and meaningless and at its worst, destructive.

Additionally, not all work creates value in monetary form. Many examples are evident: the teacher, missionary, volunteer, artist, parent, or helpful friend don't always get paid in money. In these instances, and in others, work creates value in the form of friendships, security, love, moral or aesthetic beauty, or through simple self-fulfillment, satisfaction, or a sense of duty or calling to a higher purpose. Still, the work is done to create value, just not always monetary or financial value.

In 2008, the US economy went through a period of crisis. Interest rates had been low for so long that an inevitable bubble arose in the housing and stock market. Aggressive equal opportunity government lending schemes, greed, a lack of financial regulation, consumer irresponsibility, risky loan packages, and unethical repackaging of mortgage-backed security derivatives each played a part in the 2008 crash as well. Many economists believe this crisis to have been the worst one since the Great Depression of the 1930s. Tens of thousands of Americans lost their homes, their jobs, and their investments savings. Since 2008, the economy has recovered, albeit tenuously, as governments across the globe have stepped in to provide liquidity and stimulate the economy.

Somewhere in the debate about what should have been done and what can be done now to prevent or manage another crisis, many seem to have lost sight of this fact- The only rational, reasonable, or noble goal of a business, or even of work itself is to create value. Many of the actors involved in the 2008 financial debacle were destroying value by knowingly taking worthless financial products, repackaging them, and selling them to unwitting buyers. These bad actors, criminals in many cases, were knowingly engaging in the destruction of value by unethically selling inflated derivatives at too high of a market price.

In the car business, they have a law to prevent dealers from selling cars they know are worthless or faulty, which is commonly called the "Lemon Law". Investors who bought mortgage backed securities bought "lemons- i.e. worthless or faulty investments", and all of us suffered a loss of value as a result, as the panic spread from the real estate mortgage market into the wider market. As far as I know, no one has been put in jail for any of this, but they should have been.

Commerce is a wonderful thing. At its best, business is simple and work is simple. Valuable goods or services are created and customers and/or clients pay for these goods and services and quality of life goes up for all parties. Entrepreneurs create, workers build and serve, savers save, and financiers support the value creation process and we as consumers and citizens are the better for it. Healthy work is work that creates value, both for the worker, the organization or business, and for the community at large.

It seems so simple, so easy, and so plain but we forget the reason we work, or should work, is to create value. Wonderful things like a tasty meal, a wonderful travel experience or technology product, and successful and fulfilling relationships are all created through valuable work. They are all created because these things are meaningful to us. To sum up this chapter on the purpose of *Healthy Work*, let me leave you with a quote about work, from one of the greatest leaders in business who ever lived:

"There is nothing quite so useless, as doing with great efficiency, something that should not be done at all." - Peter F. Drucker

3

What is the Responsibility of a Business?

To Create Value & Do No Harm

"There is only one ethics, one set of rules of morality, one code: That of individual behavior in which the same rules apply to everyone alike."
- Peter Drucker

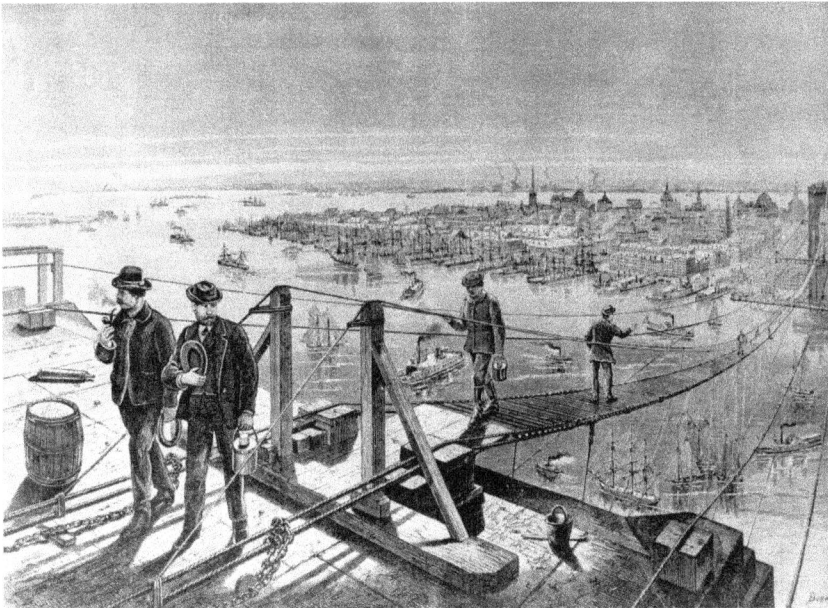

Workers on Brooklyn Bridge, New York City

D oes the name Kenneth Lay ring a bell? Kenneth Lay was the CEO of ENRON, the disgraced American energy, commodities, and financial services company found to be defrauding consumers and investors out of billions of dollars when it filed for bankruptcy in 2001. Before bankruptcy ENRON had approximately 20,000 staff members and was one of the world's largest corporations with claimed revenues of nearly $111 billion dollars. At the end of 2001, it was discovered the company's sizable financial position was sustained predominately through institutionalized, methodical, and creatively planned accounting fraud. The subsequent implosion even took down the famed accounting company *Arthur Anderson*, who had been involved in the company's accounting schemes. In a cruel case of irony, Fortune magazine named ENRON "America's Most Innovative Company" for six consecutive years. (2)

It is the responsibility of every business to be honest. This is not rocket science. Honesty is telling the truth in every way possible, to investors, employees, consumers, and the government. Trade secrets which might damage a company's competitive advantage and which are ethically held private are of course an exception. When it comes to honesty and business ethics, *transparency* is a key idea, and transparency to investors and regulators is a primary concern. Debt, profits, revenues, and all relevant accounting data should be objectively and openly detailed and reported. This is a crucial part of *Healthy Work* because unethical work is not healthy.

Governments play a key role in regulating business activity and legality. Without government regulations, businesses would undoubtedly be tempted to "cross the line" of ethics. In recent years, business schools in America have pushed the idea that businesses have an obligation to participate in society and contribute to a greater good. MBA programs now almost always require courses on ethics, leadership, and community responsibility.

Though the idea that a business has a duty to be a socially responsible and involved corporate citizen is a somewhat ambiguous and amorphous ideal, it is still a sound one, and I support this concept wholeheartedly, though individual employees should have the right to voice and disagree respectfully with their owners, managers, or fellow employees and be able to refrain from engaging in activities which conflict with their own moral, religious, and ethical code. The bottom line is that a business has a responsibility to create value and work in an honest, ethical, and legal way.

Where I live in Atlanta, GA, I have access to many questionable activities within a short driving distance. It's not directly up to me to decide whether these businesses should or should not be available to residents in my area, it's up to the local government. Smoking cigarettes, blowing money at strip clubs, eating fatty junk food, drinking excessively, playing poker, or racking up piles of debt at shopping malls may not be good for anyone, but we as free Americans have the right to do these things. The freedom to do them doesn't make them right, healthy, or good, but they are available nonetheless. Culture does affect the quality of life and health of a particular place, but the laws of our land allow us individual freedom of expression and consumption, as well as local control of business zoning and restrictions.

Practically any business product or service can hurt someone. A chiropractic adjustment could injure, a meal with bacteria could poison, or an appliance faultily wired could catch on fire. The list goes on. Our system is a system of checks and balances:

- *Businesses* should regulate *themselves*.

- *Governments* should reasonably regulate *businesses*.

- *Consumers* should *beware* of the products and services they buy.

If necessary, in cases of deliberate mistreatment of consumers or investors, legal retribution through the courts may be warranted. Sure, firearms, too much alcohol, debt, or sugar could be bad but these things can be a net good in life, if used responsibly, so we're not going to ban them. Should we put a tax on grandma's peach cobbler because it has too much sugar or fat? It's not up to a business to determine how or to what ends a consumer uses a product or service. A customer must be responsible for his own behavior. After all, a knife could be used to kill, but a knife is an indispensable part of life. We want to live in a free world with free markets, where people decide what makes them happy, but business still must always abide by Peter Drucker's admonition to lead by *"doing the right things."*

Doing the right thing and doing no harm is healthy work. In response to government pressures to reduce carbon emissions, automobile manufactures signed on and agreed to create more fuel-efficient vehicles. These ongoing efforts since the 1970s have significantly reduced pollution and smog in American cities. Whether you agree with climate change regulation or not, or pollution standards or not, it is the responsibility of businesses to follow the law. Volkswagen (VW), the iconic German car manufacturer who also owns the Audi brand, was recently exposed as having implanted a sensor into their car engines which would allow the engine to "know" when it was being tested in a lab setting, so that the engine could skirt by emission standards.

"We've totally screwed up," said VW America boss Michael Horn, while the group's chief executive at the time, Martin Winterkorn, said his company had "broken the trust of our customers and the public." Because of this ethical lapse, the company, investors, and consumers will all be damaged by these actions, which is referred to popularly as the "diesel dupe." (3) Chalk another company up on the dust heap of disgraced brands in corporate history. Companies and business people should tell the truth. Radical honesty is the only way.

In medicine, ἐπὶ δηλήσει δὲ καὶ ἀδικίῃ εἴρξειν in Greek, or *primum non nocere* in Latin, means *"first, do no harm"* and refers to the originally Greek Hippocratic Oath, thought of as the guiding ethical principle of medicine. Why not use this guiding principle in business too? I propose we operate in our working lives in the same way - do no harm.

We live in a new era. The internet and technology are ubiquitous and found in every household and in every hand in the form of a smartphone. Information about products and services is easily obtained at any time. Bad corporate news goes viral quickly. For a business model to be sustainable over the long haul in the modern technological age, a race to the top is in order, not a race to the bottom. What is best for everyone? What is the best way to create value along the value chain, in an ethical way? These are the questions every business should ask and this provides a framework in which to operate responsibly and healthily.

Disgraced investor Bernie Madoff, serving a life sentence for defrauding clients out of millions of dollars in a Ponzi scheme said, *"The nature of any human being, certainly anyone on Wall Street, is 'the better deal you give the customer, the worse deal it is for you'."*(4) Apparently, Madoff's philosophy is "heads I win, tails you lose." I couldn't disagree with Mr. Madoff's horrific "win-lose" dichotomy more. How about, as Stephen Covey wrote in his classic business book *"The 7 Habits of Highly Effective People"* we think in terms of *win-win* instead.

With healthy work, everyone wins because value is created. You win, I win, and we win. When value is created in a healthy and ethical way, all parties are the better for it.

"Character is the only way to sustain success." - John C. Maxwell

4

—

What is Healthy Work?
Meaningful & Constructive Life - Sustaining Work

"Deprived of meaningful work, men and women lose their reason for existence; they go stark raving mad."

– Fyodor Dostoevsky

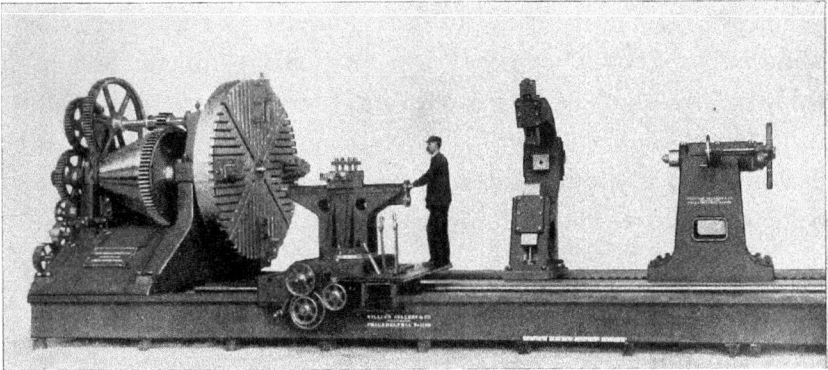

Machine Tools, 1899

H ealth is more than just the absence of disease. Health could be defined in a practical way as *a reason for being*. The Japanese have a word for this, *Ikigai*. Healthy work, using this broader definition of health, implies that our work gives us a reason to get up in the morning, an Ikigai, and is a constructive part of our life. Work can give our lives a positive meaning. Not all work is healthy. For example, crime, terrorism, or the work required to sell drugs is not healthy. Work that is destructive to oneself or others, or conflicts with positive core values is not healthy. To sum it up, healthy work builds up life and is meaningful, so....

Our goal in "Healthy Work", should be to find work that is:

• *Meaningful* and

• *Builds up* and *sustains life*, and is *constructive*.

Healthy work has integrity, and sustains and builds up life- in individuals, families, and communities, and means something. Work without meaning is like a road that leads to nowhere. If something is meaningless, it isn't healthy or unhealthy because it has no meaning. When we work to provide for our family, or for ourselves, for a cause we care about, or even for a momentary impulse to buy or enjoy a pleasurable experience, work is meaningful and healthy. Motivations change and vary. There are many ways for work to be healthy, if it is meaningful and meets the second requirement of being constructive and building up life instead of tearing it down.

For most of human history, work has been about survival. Just for the last few hundred years has prosperity reached a point where many people live lives of relative ease and where human survival is a given. Even so, there are many in developed and prosperous countries who still struggle financially, and for them work is still mainly about survival and this is the primary meaning of work, and probably always will be. Putting food on the table, paying the bills, and obtaining health care is plenty meaningful enough to many people, even in wealthy countries.

Some may attach significance to the actual craftsmanship of work, the mental and physical act of work itself, which can be rewarding and joyful. Some may have an end financial goal in mind in their efforts, so the work becomes healthy in this way. Regardless, meaningful work is healthy because it's motivating and gives us a goal to focus our minds, wills, and effort on and it strengthens our spirit. Meaning is the spark that sets the fire of work in motion and sustains the life of work. Work that has no meaning cannot by its very nature strengthen our spirit or sustain us and our life, because this type of work has no basis in the connection between cause and effect. Work without meaning is dead.

When I was a child my parents bought me a set of books on various virtues, such as discipline, character, honesty, and other values. Each book would tell the story of certain famous person in history, such as George Washington, or Louis Pasteur, or Martin Luther King Jr. and the book would describe a character trait the featured person was particularly known for, and how we should try to emulate that character trait in our lives. Though I've often fallen short of the values upheld in these books at times, they had a positive impact on me and my working life nonetheless.

One particularly healthy way to look at work is to look at work as an opportunity to build character and virtue. This is only one way to approach work, but it is a worthy way because it is self-validating. For instance, if you choose to work to become more self-disciplined or skilled in your trade, and this is your primary way of finding meaning in your work, no one can take this away from you. This internal motivation towards growth and personal development will sustain you when your work gets hard. Character driven work is its own reward.

In an interview with popular podcast host Tim Ferris, 4- Star US Army General Stanley McChristal (a man US Defense Secretary Robert Gates called *"perhaps the finest warrior and leader of men in combat I (have) ever met"*, McChristal said that in order to apply the lessons he learned in successfully serving in the military for many years, workers should overcome fear by doing what scares them. This comment from McChristal emphasizes work which centers on character growth, in this specific case overcoming fears. Development of character is only one way to approach finding meaning in work but it's particularly relevant in the modern age of technological and social upheaval. Our working life may be transient and unpredictable, but we can always focus on the self-validating aspect of character growth in our working lives, no matter what changes are taking place in the world around us.

General McChristal's concept of character work fits well with what the renowned psychiatrist Dr. Scott Peck taught in his iconic work "*The Road Less Traveled*"- life inevitably gives us problems. We can work through these life problems and become stronger or we can avoid them and let them become bigger problems. The road less traveled is about taking on challenges and growing and becoming stronger. Work can be looked at as one among many problems we'll have to solve in our lives. If we avoid the challenges that our work can bring us, we're missing an opportunity for growth. The main point is to one way or another find meaning through work, and the motivation and health that comes with it.

Regardless of your anthropological or evolutionary outlook, our primitive ancestors moved and worked to survive. This we know for certain. Sometime later, as man moved into a more settled and civilized state, he learned to farm and to store value in the form of coins, precious metals, or other types of money or valuable goods. Trade began and economic progress continued. Prosperity came to humans slowly over time from trade, knowledge, and technology, but as man worked to create value and fulfill his survival needs, and later his desires as a consumer, meaning was a given. Man worked to accomplish his various purposes and in this he attached meaning to his work.

As society progressed, trades and crafts became more specialized. Henry Ford and other inventors like Thomas Edison, or James

Watt, who invented the steam engine, were revolutionary in establishing the capitalist economy which helped to foster the economic conditions for increasing wealth dramatically and establishing a large middle class. Adam Smith discovered what made nations financially successful and wrote about it in *"The Wealth of Nations"* and later in *"A Theory of Moral Sentiments"* he expounded on what was required for a society to make capitalism work for the common good. Industry developed further in the 19th and 20th centuries as did man's appetite for consumption.

Now in modern America we live in a consumption economy. This means that our working lives are based around making money to buy more and more material goods and services to consume, most of which we don't really "need". Some men and some women work to participate as much as possible in this consumption economy and some opt for a simpler lifestyle. Not everyone is driven to buy more and more stuff. Most fall somewhere in between minimalism and high consumption.

Work done mainly for acquiring consumer goods, though common and understandable, can potentially be troublesome because trying to consume your way to happiness can be a black hole that never ends. No one can answer the question of *how much is enough?* If we spend our whole life working to buy more stuff and status with no end in sight, research shows we might end up miserable.

Work done for hierarchal rank, social status, or for accumulation of status symbols can be a trap of more debt, more stress, and a gnawing and persistent dissatisfaction with what we already have. In fact, a man can spend his entire life working for things he doesn't really want in the first place, simply because he is being manipulated by outside social forces he's not aware of. The marketing gurus of the modern consumption economy know this and they know how to push our buttons and instigate these insatiable desires.

The sociologist Max Weber illustrated this in his metaphor of the "Iron Cage", where he develops the concept of the modern man, working within the confines of a bureaucratic organization and unclear why he is working, what he is working for, or what he's even doing with his life, or for that matter who he really is, spinning his wheels alone inside the "iron cage", grasping at the ladder of hierarchal progress or for the accumulation of fleeting status symbols. Maybe he will be among the minority promoted within the cage, maybe he won't. Regardless, his work often becomes an abstraction, isolated and disconnected from his deepest values.

Sometimes, it's better to think small. Instead of getting caught in a trap where your work and consumption habits consume you, it's better to think about how you can make your working life meaningful and constructive. Avoid the pitfall of thinking you are not enough, don't have enough, or that you can't buy enough. Try thinking small.

Small is Beautiful is the title of a business book by E.F. Schumacher called *Small is Beautiful: Economics as if People Mattered*. It's good to have big goals and to dream but this book's thesis, if followed, offers a hopeful opportunity to find meaningful healthy work through smaller organizations, teams, goals, and projects. Small is often better, because even big dreams need to be broken down into smaller projects.

Thinking small allows us to find rewarding and healthy work because it allows to take on a project mindset. Projects are often more manageable than lofty and loosely defined dreams. Thinking small also gives us more control over our own working lives, particularly if we work for someone else because it gives us the space to finish things, complete tasks, and achieve goals, project by project, one day at a time.

Thinking small, we set out to learn a skill, develop a character trait, or complete a specific project at work. This happens within a positive closed feedback loop where we constantly push ourselves to improve and produce good work. Ironically, technology and the accumulation and democratization of knowledge has made this approach much more feasible to the masses in the developed world. Anyone can participate in the "small is beautiful" approach. For example, the trainer or therapist can organize his systems better in online cloud spreadsheets, restaurants and photographers can market for free using social media, a local baker can stay in touch with customers using an email chain, and the community bank can conduct business online, reducing in-person salary costs.

Technology and the information age have had a significant effect in destabilizing the bureaucratic structures of old, whether it be the state or the corporation- those of Weber's "Iron Cage", though these often leviathan organizations still play a dominant role in our society. It is now possible for every single man or woman to use technology to improve his lot in life. We are moving towards an economy in which an increasing number of people will be self-employed. The laptop is a type of factory in the modern era and the internet makes knowledge and education available to all who seek it, though there are no guarantees that anywhere close to a majority will.

Ironically, as a matter of fact, with the growth of technology's reach over time, the financial and well-being gap between those who work with drive, focus, rationality, and clear goals in mind and those who don't may grow even larger, because those with the talent, will, connections, and resources to succeed may be able to leverage these modern technological tools to an even greater degree of economic success and social collaboration and organization. Technology is available for all to use, and some are using it well, but many more are being left behind. Instead of using technology to enhance their ability to create value in the marketplace, many are becoming addicted to social media and online shopping, and some don't have access to high-tech products in the first place.

Those who use technology successfully often become even more successful and self-selective geographically and socially, based on their rising economic status. We should, as thoughtful and empathetic citizens, take this into account as we witness a type of technology-driven Darwinism play itself out in the marketplace of labor and some workers are left behind. Despite the downsides though, many who come from underprivileged or rudimentary backgrounds have indeed used technology to leverage their unique skills and talents to find life-sustaining health and constructive meaning in their work. Generations ago, these modern entrepreneurs and enterprising workers may have been stuck pushing a plow, standing on an assembly line all day, or raising an army of farmhands, all noble and good work, but often much more grueling and less rewarding than the self-directed work they're engaged in today. The jury is still out on where technology and the so-called "knowledge revolution" will lead us but it has been a positive game-changer for many.

Seasons of work come and go like the seasons of nature. Sometimes work is confusing, we feel lost, or we're just not motivated. We know it's good to work. We like making money, need to work, and we value work on a material, moral, ethical, and social level, but other than that we're aren't sure what we're working for. Periods of time like this could be viewed as a *season* of work, like a season of nature. Winter is cold, dark, and dead, and at times our work may feel this way as well. Little meaning can seem to be found in the "winters" of work.

This is perfectly normal and even can be a chance for us to explore, make new connections, try new things, and have new work experiences. We might decide to volunteer, or take on a unique project we've never done, just for the sake of the experience. This type of exploratory work can be healthy too. We can start to learn more about ourselves, what type of work we enjoy or don't enjoy, and we can just enjoy the process of learning more about ourselves and what we're good at.

The *Harvard Business Review* offers some solid advice for those who are at a crossroads in work and looking for a different direction: In an older paradigm, the model for a career was to "plan & implement" but with the changes going on in the world of work it might be necessary to engage in a strategy of "test & learn" instead (5). Try new things, experiment, volunteer in your spare time, take a class, take on challenging assignments, look for new connections between people, places, or skills. See where this exploration leads you. On the path to healthy work, don't be afraid to try new things.

Work should be meaningful for it to be healthy. Just supporting yourself, and your family if you have one, is plenty good and meaningful enough to have a healthy working life. The meaning behind your work may change often over a lifetime. Work done responsibly and with an effort to create value, sustain life, and not hurt anyone is a good thing and an undeniably admirable pursuit, whatever it might be.

"Being the richest man in the cemetery doesn't matter to me. Going to bed at night saying we've done something wonderful, that's what matters to me." -Steve Jobs

5

—

What are the Values of Healthy Work?

The Characteristics of Work That Make It Healthy and Life-Sustaining

"The good of man is a working of the soul in the way of excellence in a complete life." –Aristotle, The Nicomachean Ethics

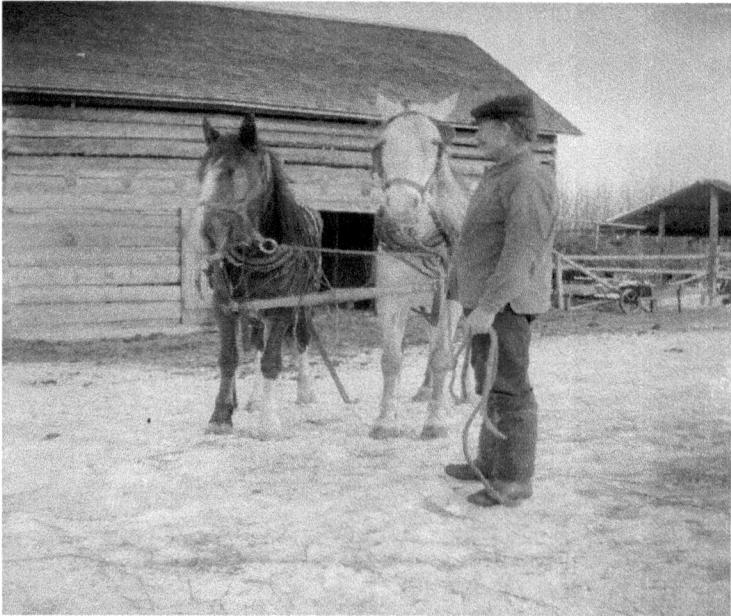

A Farmer & His Horses, 1900

healthy work

I have been fortunate enough to travel to over 30 countries on 6 Continents. I've noticed, observed, and studied one phenomena which stands out. Americans who work spend more hours working than workers do in most any other country. Most American workers have 2 or 3 weeks of time off every year at the most. From 18 to roughly 70 years of age or so, most Americans will be working 40-60 hours per week and we are known worldwide for being workaholics. Since we spend so much of our lives working, we should decide what we value the most about work, and which values will make our working lives healthy.

We've established thus far in the previous chapters:

- Work is good

- Work is done to create value and fulfill human needs and desires.

- Work's responsibility is to be valuable and to do no harm.

- Work done in a healthy way is meaningful, constructive, and builds or sustains life.

This next question should then be asked: What are the values of healthy work? In other words, what should we value about work, those traits which make work healthy? The following list is not the entire spectrum of good values for work, but they're a good start. They'll get you thinking more about valuing the right things in your working life. Instead of diving into a long and drawn out philosophical explanation of each working value, the nature of each in a work environment will be examined in a case study format. You could write an entire book on each value if you wanted to, but we'll keep it short.

It's a good idea to decide ahead of time to deliberately live out our core values in our chosen work. Harvard Business School professor Dr. Clay Christensen, in his inspirational and timely book *How Will You Measure Your Life?* writes about his former business students' values and how their lives turned out: *"I know for sure that none of these people graduated with a deliberate strategy to get divorced or lose touch with their children—much less to end up in jail. Yet this is the exact strategy that too many ended up implementing."* Christensen teaches that we should emphasize our life resources, and how we use them- *time, money, and relationships.* Are we valuing the right things? What we value most can be seen by the way we live and the way we work, not by what we say.

I've chosen my top 8 core values in my own business and work, because they are self-validating, meaning they are good things regardless of how much money is made or how much worldly success is attained. You may choose different values as your guiding principles, so these are only examples. I try to always live up to my core values, though it's easy to get off course and fall short at times.

Ethical

Recent cases of tobacco companies being forced to pay out billions of dollars in fines and settlements in negligence cases could have been avoided, had the companies acted in an ethical manner. Had they been honest and up front about the negative health consequences of tobacco, they probably wouldn't have been sued. Being ethical means being honest, and following the rules and laws of a given community. The dictionary defines ethics as: *that branch of philosophy dealing with values relating to human conduct, with respect to the rightness and wrongness of certain actions and to the goodness and badness of the motives and ends of such actions.* Tobacco should be legal and available, but companies should not try to cover up the fact that it's harmful. There's nothing wrong with selling tobacco, but pretending its not unhealthy is unethical and wrong. Ethical work is healthy work, because it brings out our highest potential.

Radically Honest

Radical honesty is a value I learned about a few years ago. It's based on the work of Dr. Brad Blanton, who wrote a book by the same name - "Radical Honesty" in 1996. Radical honesty stands in contrast to plain-old-fashioned honesty in that it seeks to go a step beyond just being honest to being courageous in telling uncomfortable truths. The benefits are trust, openness, intimacy, and authentic connection. Honesty takes courage and vulnerability, and radical honesty takes even more.

In my own work of personal training, wellness coaching, and counseling people on nutritional and other health issues, I came to the realization that for the first part of my career I was only honest in my practice, not *radically honest*. This held me back, in the sense that I would tell people at times what they wanted to hear. I made good connections and had close relationships but they were not as authentic as they could have been. When I started to highly value and employ radical honesty, I lost some clients and probably some friends, but I have made even stronger bonds with customers, clients, and friends. Radical honesty might sound harsh or extreme but it is the best way to live because it implies a strong boundary of truthfulness.

Caring

Work should be done with care-for the work, the worker, the employer, the community, and the customer. Work done in any other way is not healthy. Peter Drucker taught that the entire purpose of a business is to create and serve a customer. Integrative and expansive caring is important and without caring about each component of work - the work itself, the worker, employer, and community- work could eventually lose meaning and become destructive. If you don't care, work gets sloppy. Products and services become subpar and care-less. The word "careless" is fitting and work should never be careless.

When I was in graduate school, I had the opportunity to work at a local YMCA in Atlanta. The YMCA is an organization which exemplifies this trait and they name caring as one of their core values. Started as a Christian based inner-city gym and lodging place for men during the Industrial Era of the late 1800s, the *Young Men's Christian Association* has always tried to live out the value of caring. Even today, YMCAs offer scholarships to underprivileged and at-risk youth.

Competitive

Competitive as an admirable value may come as a surprise to some. Competition has been given a bad name by political correctness. In the effort to create a more equal society, the cultural emphasis on competition has been de-emphasized in the name of equality, so that often no one wins or loses, or stands out, and "everyone gets a trophy". This is not good. Winning and losing is part of life. In some ways, life will always be a competition, if not with others then with ourselves. Competition makes work meaningful and healthy because competition in its most pure and ethical form is about character development.

When we compete, we are not literally trying to eliminate the other competitor, at least not in the post--industrial age. We can think *win-win* when we compete, instead of *win-lose*. In a lodestar of a business book, *Understanding Michael Porter*, the thesis is put forth based on Michael Porter's research and work at Harvard Business School that the way to create winning value in modern business, considering the effect of technology and the internet, is to compete by being unique and finding a competitive advantage, not necessarily by beating the other business.

Microsoft and Apple can both be successful and survive, but they must each do what they do uniquely the best and do it the best they can. In other words, they need to focus on competing with themselves by trying to get better at what they do, instead of trying to eliminate the other. Even in the field of sports, titans like legendary football coach Vince Lombardi and current superstar coach Nick Saban are ferociously committed to coaching basic techniques and fundamentals, which is much the same idea: Compete with yourself to be the best you can be to win. Who you become "in the process" as Nick Saban says is as important as the scoreboard.

Goal-Oriented

In the industrial era, workers could afford to show up and be told what to do. Those days are over. In a large sense, we're going back to the pre-industrial era where initiative will be required in our labor. Modern work should be built around goals and more specifically projects. In his inspiring and insightful book *Lynchpin,* Seth Godin writes eloquently of the need for modern workers to view themselves as a "lynchpin", an essential part of the team, without which tremendous loss would be felt within an organization, even if it is a large company.

In other words, work should always have a specific goal or project in mind to create value. Every worker should have goals. We should set goals, define projects, put ourselves out there, and not be afraid to show our work to the world. The days of hiding are over. Seth Godin also refers to this as "shipping"- creating something of value and putting it out there for the world to see. Another way this has been put, in the outstanding personal development and business book *"The Freaks Shall Inherit the Earth"* is:

1) Make a plan.

2) Stick to it.

3) If you don't have a plan, make one.

Disciplined

We will all experience one of two things: the pain of discipline, or the pain of regret.

- Jim Rohn

I have a friend Robert who eats the same thing for breakfast every day. He also wears a white dress shirt every day to work with a blue suit. He occasionally wears a red tie, or a blue one, or a black one. He also exercises every day, and doesn't drink during the week. He goes to church every Sunday and never cheats on his wife. He is a happy and successful person who has contributed much to the community and done meaningful work. Why has he been able to achieve this? My friend, who is a former military officer, is one of the most successful and disciplined people I've ever met.

Time after time, discipline keeps coming up as one of the most important values we can have when it comes to work, particularly since work is becoming increasingly self-directed. Discipline is the heart and soul of keeping the work train running. Steve Jobs wore the same black turtleneck most of the time, and only had a handful of items of clothing. This freed Jobs up to work on other more important things, and with what he did in his working life with Apple, well the rest is history. Jobs was a discipline machine.

Discipline is irreplaceable and foundational for healthy work, but luckily, it's like a "muscle" which can be built over time. You don't need to be a minimalist like Steve Jobs or my successful friend I wrote about but you do need to do it when you don't want to do it. Never forget: movement is motivation. Don't wait for some magical feeling of motivation. You may never want to do it but you must do it anyway. Without doing things we "don't feel like doing", over and over in a disciplined way, nothing will get done!

Courageous

Courageous people do courageous things. As stated previously, the days of showing up and getting by are over and done with. Mankind in his primitive state had to think creatively, to ward off predators, to wall of the perimeters, and to hunt, build, and survive. Our ancestors had to be courageous just to survive. The labor required of us now in modern times will once again require us to be more courageous, at least emotionally, if not physically.

We may have to go search for new work, change careers, form alliances, create our own businesses, or speak up in our current work environments. The point is, the status quo is no longer good enough. The bad news is that those who aren't courageous or disciplined may be left to whine and complain, or protest for an easier way, or lobby for government bailouts or a sinecure. Some will need time to become courageous, and we should care for them, be patient with them, and urge them along to a new way of looking at work. Who exemplifies courageous work better than the civil rights leaders like MLK Jr. or a founding father like Benjamin Franklin, George Washington, or Thomas Jefferson, who died working in the case of MLK, or could have become a martyr in the case of Franklin, Washington, or Jefferson? Each was willing to be courageous to the point of death to do the job. That's healthy work.

Self-Validated

As discussed in the chapter on meaningful work, self-validation is something which should be valued highly in work. Work which fits with our highest ideals, ethics, and morals, is work which is valuable internally and should give us joy. Some workers, such as the writer John Kennedy Toole, create prized masterpieces such as his book *"A Confederacy of Dunces"* which later won the Pulitzer Prize after Toole's suicidal death, but they are not able to experience the joy of their efforts. This is a tragedy. We should take immense pleasure in doing a good job.

Some people work and then sadly can't see the beauty in their own creation, the courage and will in it, and suffer as a result. Others can tap into this valuable insight of self-validation and experience work in this way. After suffering and witnessing unspeakable horrors as a prisoner in Nazi death camps, Viktor Frankl said, *"Everything can be taken from a man but one thing: the last of the human freedoms—to choose one's attitude in any given set of circumstances, to choose one's own way."* Frankl came to the realization that no one could rob him of his dignity and that he could work to do what he could, to live and find meaning in the hand that he had been dealt.

Even in tragedy, healthy work can be done within ourselves. Valuing the right things in our working lives makes work healthy. At certain times in life, it's good to take a step back and ask, what do I value most? When a person looks at his work, what does he want to see in it looking back at him? These are the values of healthy work, the things that give our work weight, and a tangible, emotional, and moral presence, and in turn make work meaningful and life-sustaining.

These values I listed, and you may add others to your list, are like road signs which point out a route and destination in our working lives. They let us know if we are getting off track and point to the things which make work healthy in the long run. That way, when the sun sets on a lifetime, we can look back at our work and be proud of what we did. Mark Twain once said, *"The fear of death follows from the fear of life. A man who lives fully is prepared to die at any time."* A man who works with values in mind is preparing himself for whatever may come, by working in the moment with integrity and purpose.

6

—

What are the Components of a Healthy Work Environment?

Integrating Mind, Body, & Spirit

"The head rules the belly through the chest. The heart is not above the head, but it can and should obey it." —CS Lewis

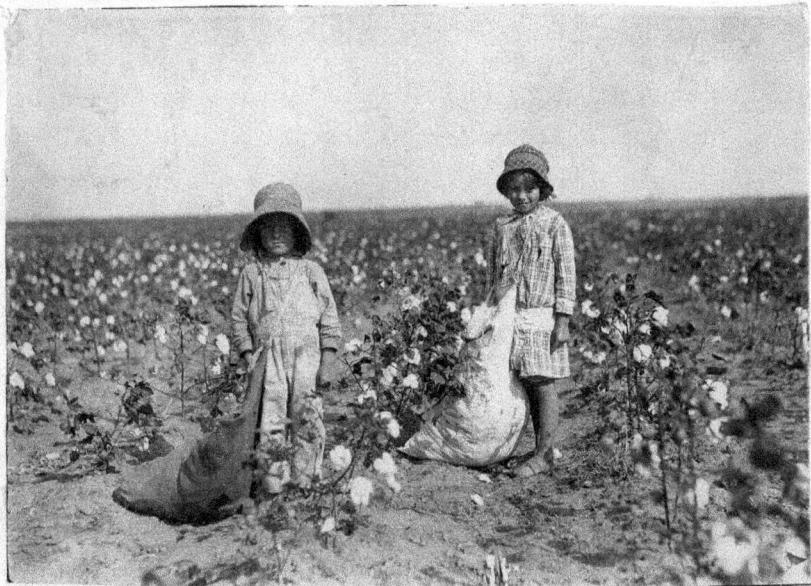

Jewel & Harold Walker Picking Cotton, 1910

Lawrence: "What would you do if you had a million dollars?
Peter: "Nothing, absolutely nothing."   *- Office Space*

And with those words the protagonist Peter Gibbons, the lead character in one of the most famous modern American cinematic comedies, *Office Space*, sums up the way many people feel about work these days. Office Space is an iconic film because it struck a cultural nerve. Work does feel meaningless to many people. We often work for corporations owned by stockholders we'll never meet, and which are run by executives and managers who often aren't loyal to the companies they work for and could care less about their employees, while we do mind-numbing and menial work. We are treated at times like cogs in a machine, because often we are. Technology has routinized many jobs to the point where people aren't needed anymore or if they are needed, they're needed much less.

Our entire economy is based largely on consumption- what people want, not what they need. To survive, all a person needs is a place to sleep, some food, and health care. Anything on top of that is up to the person. People want different things. In my book, *Movement & Meaning: Building Mental Strength and Managing Stress through Exercise,* I went to great lengths to describe in detail how stressed out and miserable people can become living a life of insatiable desire for material goods and experiences. Again, this is like Max Weber's analogy of the *Iron Cage*, or the "Ring" in *The Lord of the Rings*, which represents the *precious, precious* ring of a never-ending circle of desperation, dissatisfaction, and despair. *Wants* aren't bad, we all have *wants*, but how we handle our wants will determine whether our work builds us up and is fulfilling, or it stresses us out and tears us down.

Then what are we to do when it comes to work? How do we bring humanity, courage, and connection back to the work environment? The industrial revolution is winding down, particularly in America, and it's time to move on. Even though we are living through volatile changes in work, society, and culture, changes which we often aren't aware of and have difficulty conceptualizing, these dramatic changes offer us a chance, if we have the courage to take it. For the first time in human history, we have the freedom to work in the best way we see fit. We aren't locked into a set path when we're born and we can choose our own way in life.

For better or worse, hierarchies and systems of social organization are breaking down. We don't have to live lives ruled by consumerism, industrial control, and mindless conformity anymore. We can instead strive for our highest mental, physical, and spiritual potential as we work. For perhaps the first time in history, most of us have a real opportunity to completely own our labor and work how we see fit. Extraordinary changes bring downsides but also extraordinary opportunity, the opportunity to create a healthy working life. Through discipline, through courage, through creativity, through the right values, and through patience we can employ the components of healthy work in our organizations and in ourselves and create a better future.

You should start to think of yourself as the CEO of "You, Inc." or the mayor of your own city. The Greek Philosopher Aristotle taught thousands of years ago that every person was like a city in miniature and his timeless advice is just as relevant today. He wisely urged us to rule our "inner city" with Justice and Virtue just as a wise ruler would rule his city. If we could master ourselves, Aristotle believed, we could create a better world. That's what *Healthy Work* is about- mastering ourselves. Work is not about doing what is easy or doing what we've always done. Healthy work is about rising to the occasion.

When I was born, I was lazy. When I was born, I had a temper. When I was born, I was selfish. When I was born, I was afraid. When I was born, I was undisciplined. When I was born, I was a child. I can still be each of those things and I fight them every day, because I don't want to be the way I was born. I want to be better than that. *Healthy work* is about being better. Healthy work is about:

- Acknowledging that work is good and valuing it in ourselves and in other people.

- Valuing the right things *about* work- caring, discipline, ethics, etc.

- Creating productive value without doing harm.

- Doing meaningful, constructive, and life-sustaining labor.

Being healthy means being healthy in mind, body, and spirit. Work should be approached the same way and should integrate our physical body, our thoughts and habits, and our spiritual desires, values, and lifetime goals.

Work should involve a healthy mind:

We should challenge ourselves to learn, to develop new skills, and to achieve goals and finish projects.

Work should involve a healthy body:

We should take care of our physical health while we're working.

Work should involve a healthy spirit:

We should care about our work and what it means and what legacy we're leaving in our work when we're gone.

These components call on us to engage our entire being in our work- our minds, bodies, and our deepest held desires and spiritual values, so that we can work in the healthiest way possible over our lifetime.

Pull out a journal and answer these questions about your work:

a. Spiritual Health

i. Purpose- Do you have a deep connection to your work? What are you working for? This can be as simple as developing greater inner character or working to support your family because you love them.

ii. Transcendence- Do you have a sense that what you do in this life matters? Can you get in touch with this through your work? Do your values and ethics match up with the work you're doing? If not, what can be changed? What will you leave behind when your work is done?

iii. Community- How is your work connected to the people in your neighborhood and city and to those who live and work near you?

iv. Family- Do you work in a way that is supportive of your family? Are you allowing your work to act in a destructive way towards your family?

b. Physical

i. Nature- How often do you see sunlight at work? Do you work in an environment where you have access to light? Natural sunlight is an oft-forgotten stimulus for Vitamin D and is very healthy. Do you have time to get outside during the work day, and get sunlight and fresh air? If not, how can you incorporate nature into your work day? It is not healthy to be indoors all the time.

iii. Activity- Do you have a chance to be active during the work day? Excessive sitting is destructive for health and many have called sitting the new smoking. If we were to design the worst possible work environment, it would be the cubicle: social isolation, no natural light, no room to move around, and excessive sitting.

iv. **Food and water-** Are healthy food and snacks available to you throughout the day? Are you avoiding high-calorie, fatigue-inducing meals? Are you hydrated, drinking 6-8 glasses of water per day? Are you avoiding sugar and the energy crashes that come with it?

v. **Noise-** Is excessive, distracting, or unnecessary noise present in the work environment? How can you eliminate noise and distraction?

c. Mental / Psychological

The hallmark of unhealthy & stressful work is *responsibility with no control.* No control over a work problem coupled with responsibility over it causes feelings of overwhelm and heavy stress, which can damage your health. In other words, if you cannot control a work situation, but you're held responsible for how it turns out, you're working in an unhealthy environment. Our brains and minds were not made to work this way. We need to find ways to specifically cope with and control our work environments as much as possible.

i. **Territory & Project Focused-** How can you think smaller? How can you develop teams in your workplace? How can you shift your work to a project orientation? Try to restructure your work in terms of smaller things you can get done. For example, I wrote this book called "Healthy Work", one day and one chapter at a time. A territory is a positive feedback loop. Planting a garden, setting up a sales pitch, walking 3 miles per day, or writing an essay are all territory-focused projects. We give and we get something back in return in a territory- peace of mind. Think small, and in this way, think about your territory and get your projects done.

ii. Cyclical- Can you push hard, take breaks, rest, celebrate small wins, and find balance in your work, living and working one hour, one day, and one week at a time?

iii. Intellectually Challenging- Is the work you're doing challenging you to think, to learn, to adapt, and to change for the better?

iv. Safe- Are you free to respectfully speak your mind in a professional way, and generally be yourself, free from harassment, intimidation, or groupthink in your work environment?

v. Productive- Are you producing finished work projects, achieving goals, and accomplishing valuable things that matter? Are you turning out quality services and finished products? Try using the *80/20 Rule*- 80% of your success comes from 20% of your efforts, and the same can be said for stress and time-wasters. 80% of the negativity and stress in your work and life probably comes from the same 20% of sources. Try to eliminate the 20% which are dragging you down and focus on the 20% which give you the most productive results.

vi. Communication- Are the other members of your work team aware of everything going on in the workplace? Do the channels of communication flow openly at work? Are you in regular contact with each of your team members?

vii. Stress- Do you have control over your work environment? How do you cope with stress at work? Are you communicating with your team about workplace challenges? How can you get more responsibility to deal with the problems that come up at work? Try learning and using stress-reduction techniques like breathing exercises, meditation, listening to music, journaling, or taking walks.

Periodically, at least once a year, review these questions. Perform an "audit" of your working life to see if it's healthy based on what you learned. If not, make some changes. If we do what we've always done, we'll get what we've always gotten. Healthy work requires doing the best we can to become better day-by-day, both mentally, physically, and spiritually.

7

What Does Healthy Work Look Like in the Real World?

Case Studies

"Self-esteem comes from achievement, not lax standards and false praise." - Condoleezza Rice

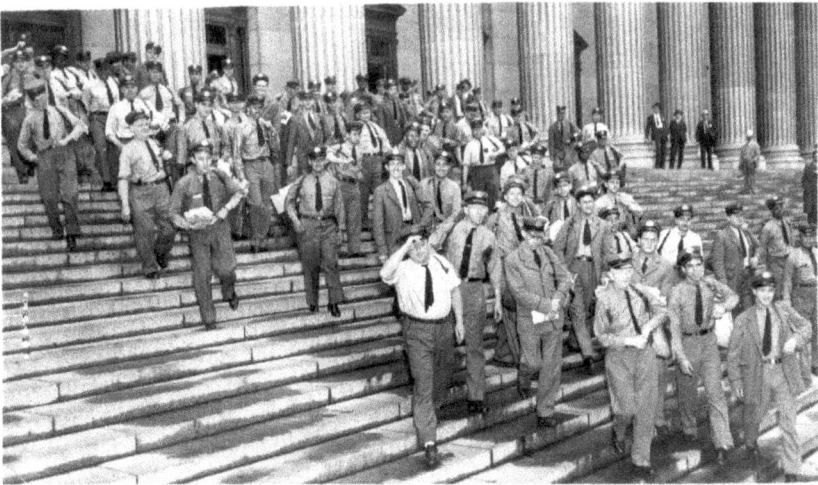

Mail Carriers Set Out, 1936

W ork - related stress is a major factor in our health, and stress itself is the number one killer in America. The number of people living alone in the US is the highest it's ever been and it's estimated that over 25% of the US population has no close friends at all. Depression is the leading cause of disability claims in the US and about 1/4 of the population struggles with mental illness at some point throughout each year. The country spends approximately *$500 billion* dollars annually on treatments related to mental illness. Men struggle with addiction and drug and alcohol abuse more than women, while women struggle with depression and anxiety more frequently. No matter how you look at it, Americans are struggling with stress, and work is part of the problem.

Both men and women are trying to understand their role and place in the new globalized economy. Many are dropping out of the workforce altogether, placing a strain on government budgets. The US deficit stood at *$18,966,715,325,873* trillion dollars and counting in 2016. Working - class middle-aged white Americans are dying faster than any other group in the country. Surveys tell us that Americans are not optimistic about the future. Wages are stagnant and have been for many years, free trade deals have de-industrialized the US economy and along with questionable social policies have combined to destabilize working families. No matter which way you spin it, something is amiss in America and the state of work has something to do with it. (6)

Though we live longer and have more cheap consumer goods than previous generations, and though the unemployment rate is low, 5-6% as of January 2016, we aren't necessarily improving our overall quality of life or health. Just because we have more material goods doesn't mean we're necessarily healthier or happier. The U.S. Declaration of Independence proclaimed "life, liberty, and the *pursuit* of happiness" as a fundamental opportunity afforded to American citizens but it never *guaranteed* we'd all be happy. Despite the US economy being the largest in the world, and despite having one of the highest per capita income rates in the world, we seem to not be getting everything right. We are unsure about the future, unsure about our country's direction, and unsure about the meaning of it all, including our work.

Many families would prefer only one parent working while they have small children, but due to many factors, they feel like they can't make it with one income so both parents work, which puts strains on marriages and families. 1/2 to 3/4 of working class children are born to unmarried parents, and research shows us these children are more likely to struggle in life in many ways. Public, religious, and civic life all have declining participation rates, highlighted extensively in the recent literary non-fiction classics *Bowling Alone* and *Coming Apart* by political scientist Charles Murray. These and other economic and social changes are contributing significantly to a workplace challenge we are persistently running into in American life more generally: moral and ethical confusion, nihilism, and a decline in social trust and social cohesion. Tellingly, affluent Americans have largely bypassed many of these social problems and maintained a lifestyle which is like more socially conservative eras of the past.

Our country is balkanized and we're having an identity crisis. Who are we? Who is right? What is right? Why should we work in the first place, if we don't have to? Why is it not ok to outsource jobs, expatriate capital gains, have many children while living on welfare without being married, pollute the environment, engage in perpetual war, sell unscrupulously, punish small business owners with bureaucratic red tape, invade consumers' privacy, or do anything else which might be considered immoral, distasteful, or unethical, if there is no such thing as a universal "good" anymore? No one has an answer to these questions.

Someone said once that America was more like a business than a country. Unfortunately, we may be seeing the fruits of that painful truth come to a head in the 2016 political season with the rise of populist anger realized in the ascendancy of Donald Trump and Bernie Sanders as the "business" of America doesn't seem to be working for many. Most Americans, though they may not know exactly what's happening, or even have the time or motivation to investigate deeply, know something isn't quite right. At the time of this book's publishing, the unthinkable has happened and Donald Trump has won the US Presidency with the backing of the rightfully angry working class.

Both political parties seem to have neglected the reinvestment this country needs in its economic and social well-being in favor of "laisse-faire" economic and social policies. The framers of the US constitution, inspired mainly by enlightenment thinkers like John Locke and David Hume, among others, and by the uniquely Christian moral sense of human dignity, set us on a path which created the strongest country in the world. But they also warned that freedom requires respect for the law, personal responsibility, and moral character. John Adams, the 2nd President of the US, once wrote: *"Our constitution was made only for a moral and religious people. It is wholly inadequate to any other."* One must ponder how Adam's thought would sit in today's postmodern age, which is wholescale rejection of any universal moral or ethical standards.

In his exceptional book, *The Righteous Mind,* liberal and democratic thinker and writer Jonathan Haidt admirably went to extraordinary lengths to bridge the political divide in the US. American citizens lean either more liberal or more conservative, but according to Haidt, we can get into trouble when we don't balance out values which work together to create a cohesive culture that works for everyone. These values, according to Haidt, are care, fairness, liberty, loyalty, authority and sanctity. Liberals tend to rate very highly on care and fairness whereas conservatives tend to rate more moderately on all 6. Either way, we should try to look at the big picture and incorporate all 6 of these values in our lives as citizens, and make the fairest and most balanced judgments we can about what is the best way to live and to work. Otherwise our working lives, and our perspective on the social world is never going to be cohesive and healthy. (7)

Healthy Work is not about politics, but *Healthy Work* is about putting the "good" back into work. Unfortunately, making a statement about what is good has become political as the country has become more partisan, multi-cultural, and polarized, because what is good to one person might not be to another. *Healthy work* is first and foremost about what is good: good for the worker, the employer, the entrepreneur, and for society and a clear step forward in the right direction. *Healthy Work* is an unintentionally polarizing but purposefully balanced assessment about what is good when it comes to work, and the best way to get there.

Let's review:

- Work is good.

- Work creates value and fulfills human needs & desires.

- Work should create real value and do no harm.

- Work should be meaningful and life-sustaining to be healthy.

- Work should integrate the mind, body, & spirit.

Case Studies

When attempting to define and promote a healthy working life it helps to look at some positive examples. Despite all the bad news out there, there are plenty of Americans who have found meaningful, fulfilling, and rewarding work, working for themselves or for someone else. Plenty of US companies are doing things the right way and many American workers have a healthy working life.

I've had interesting jobs in my life. I got my first job when I was 14, going door-to-door in the neighborhood to ask neighbors if I could help them with yard work. Technically I had been working since I was younger, helping around the house and helping my Dad in the yard and on the house. Later I worked at Taco Bell, K-Mart, Hardees, Little Caesar's Pizza, as a lifeguard, at a local gym, doing construction, at Maples Industries in the Maintenance Department, Chuck's BBQ, the Student Activities Center at Auburn University, and at the YMCA, before graduating from graduate school in Atlanta and starting my own business. Along the way, I did other odd jobs here and there also.

My early work experience was invaluable. I learned to be empathetic with people who are working jobs which are not glamorous and in which they deal with a lot of headaches for low wages. I also learned that I was motivated to go to college so I could hopefully do work which more interesting and meaningful to me, and frankly so I wouldn't have to have a job I hated my whole life. I also learned that I needed to become more motivated and disciplined because I was not that way naturally, but regardless I always enjoyed working.

Of all the work I've done, I enjoyed working at Chuck's BBQ in Auburn, AL the best, other than my current business. This job which I held from ages 19-20, where I eventually became an assistant manager, allowed me independence at work and allowed me to learn about customer service and about taking initiative. I was still immature at the time, but I enjoyed the fact that it was a small business and that I knew the owner well and he seemed to care about me. To me this sense of being cared for made a big difference in how I viewed the work. I felt cared for, so I cared more about the work. In the following paragraphs, I've selected 4 companies which I admire as case studies in *Healthy Work* based on the values I laid out in earlier chapters. There are of course many other companies which could have been chosen but one thing the following have in common is that they treat their employees like family.

I am a supporter of free markets. Through extensive study of government and history, as well as what I've learned from traveling all over the world and seeing different economic and political systems in action, I strongly prefer imperfect capitalism over any other system. The evidence clearly says it works the best for all parties involved in creating a peaceful and prosperous society. Capitalism isn't a perfect system, particularly if the legal and political system is corrupt. So, we need the rule of law to make sure capitalism happens in a just way. Just as important, less advantaged and talented citizens in our communities can get left behind as the economically and intellectually successful self-segregate geographically and socially year after year, extrapolating out eventually into a divided nation engaged in a winner-take-all survival of the fittest. We should remember the ones who get left behind by capitalism.

My own work philosophy is one I would call "community capitalism" or "localist" where judgements are made, and standards, expectations, and boundaries are enforced, but at the end of the day there is a sense of transcendent purpose and where extensive patience and kindness is shown in the work environment, including in the immediate geographical community. With the tumult and upheaval in the US economic and social world, work should be a refuge, a place which brings out the best in everyone and allows growth, belonging, contribution, integrity and thus, *Healthy Work*.

The following are 4 companies which I admire, and which in my estimation uphold the values laid out in this book.

Patagonia

When I first read the story of Patagonia, it struck a nerve with me because I love the outdoors. Patagonia is iconic company which offers employees a sense of belonging and purpose connected to the natural world. The founder, Yvon Chouinard, got his start in small business making rock climbing equipment and eventually founded the outdoor equipment and clothing company. Chouinard committed from the beginning to make Patagonia a fantastic place to work and as an avowed environmentalist he attracted talented employees and partners who shared his worldview and wanted to work for a company which supported environmental causes. Some perks include company "tithing" for environmental activism and paying employees to take breaks and work on local environmental projects. Patagonia also switched to using all organic cotton when research showed that it was better for the environment.

Many Americans don't share the same concerns for the environment that Patagonia does, but that's not the point. Patagonia does work which is connected to bigger things, like the health of the natural ecosystem, and there are plenty of talented workers who want to work for a company like that. Being branded as a company which cares about the environment certainly helps sales as well. Though the company is set up as a private "B Corp", or public benefit corporation, and doesn't issue common stock, it brought in over $600 million dollars in sales in 2016 and is growing fast. As CEO Rose Marcario said recently in a Fast Company interview, *"You can't really split your working life from the life you live every day as a person."*

Chick-fil-A

Chick-fil-A is closed on Sundays. Anyone who is from Georgia where the quickly growing restaurant chain started could tell you that. Because closing on Sunday is such a rare thing in the non-stop, 24/7, cutthroat business market of the US, the company's focus on family values and care for employees and customers, and for simply taking a day of rest, has helped make it extremely popular in the conservative Southern US and beyond. Any visit to the chain will bring you 3 consistent things: 1) Cleanliness 2) Good food & 3) Polite and considerate service.

I know several Special Olympic athletes who have had jobs at Chick-fil-A and I can tell you from experience that this company has an unparalleled culture of doing things the right way. My great aunt knew the Cathy family, who started Chick-fil-A, and they went to church together for many years at Jonesboro Baptist Church in Georgia. When my aunt passed away, the Cathy family sent Chick-fil-A chicken nuggets to the house for the wake.

In an age of hedge funds and corporations sweeping in to lay off 2000 employees just before Christmas to save a few bucks, this company is a breath of fresh air. Chick-fil-A demonstrates *Healthy Work* because they treat their employees and customers with dignity, expecting the best from their workers, but caring about their wellbeing and quality of life. Though the company's official slogan is *"We didn't invent the chicken, just the chicken sandwich"*, their unofficial motto seems to be - doing things the right way, inside the store and out.

Lodge Cast Iron

The National Cornbread Festival, which involves a cornbread eating contest, a beauty pageant, and a cornbread cooking competition, takes place in South Pittsburgh, TN annually. I've been several times and it's always a blast. The festival was the brainchild of the Lodge family, owners of the *Lodge Cast Iron Co.* since the 19th century. The company started as a small foundry in 1896 and has since ebbed and flowed but has maintained its presence as one of the biggest employers in South Pittsburgh (pop. 3000) and Marion County, TN. To many, *cast-iron* is synonymous with southern cooking and with Appalachia, so with the recent resurgence of interest in local cooking, the company has taken off once again with higher sales. Still, the company has not forgotten its roots or connections to the small TN town of 20 churches, 2 bars, a Wal-Mart (the biggest employer) and a moderately busy main street.

There was a time in American life when most businesses were owned by local citizens. Owners invested profits back into the communities they lived in. Owners and citizens lived together, worked together, worshipped together, and played together. Though financial derivatives and common ownership of public corporations have created great wealth for a small minority of Americans, it has a come at a cost. The type of community fostered by companies like *Lodge* has been lost to a large degree.

Lodge is a unique case of *Healthy Work* because of its emphasis on being an integral part of the local community. It is not an anonymous and amorphous multi-national corporation as so many US companies have become. Many people in America are anonymous- at home, in their neighborhood, at work, and everywhere else they go. Many people come and go to work without any connection to the city or community they work in, which is not a healthy way to work. Atlanta author and businessman Sam Williams addressed the possible positive and negative outcomes of this anonymity in his book, *CEO as Urban Statesman*, when he discussed the powerful change agent business leaders can be for good when they get involved in local community issues. (8) Oftentimes though, business leaders, particularly those at the helm of behemoth multinationals, choose to ignore local community concerns to significant detriment.

Lodge is only a small company, and I'm biased in my affection for Lodge because I grew up 30 minutes from South Pittsburgh and because I love cornbread and cast iron cooking, but it's an organization I admire. They are pivotal part of their local community, enriching the working lives of many people. Working Americans need more than a TV to watch at night, a smartphone to stare at, and a beer to drink. They should be proud of the company they work for and the work they do. Workers need to be part of a community, and part of a larger story that matters. *Healthy Work* involves caring and creating value, through the products and services being sold, and through the investment in the surrounding community.

The Ritz Carlton Hotels

Creating a healthy company involves creating a work culture based on integrity which team members can get behind. Hiring the right people, who want to treat the customer right from the day they're hired and who want to be a part of a winning team, is what sets *The Ritz Carlton Hotels* apart. *"Ladies and Gentlemen serving Ladies & Gentlemen"* is the motto put in place by Horst Schulze, who I once saw speak at the Buckhead Rotary Club about his long and inspirational tenure as President of the company. In an interview with Forbes magazine in 2012 Schulze said:

"We are superior to the competition because we hire employees who work in an environment of belonging and purpose. That is my mantra. We foster a climate where the employee can deliver what the customer wants. You cannot deliver what the customer wants by controlling the employee. Employees who are controlled cannot respond caringly, you need superior knowledge and real leadership, not management. Because of this we specifically developed a selection process for leaders; we don't hire managers.

The finest people in the world work in our hotels and I don't let just somebody train them when we open a hotel, I train them. I did that in 50 Ritz Carltons and I still do it. I do it because I love it, not because I have to.

I'll give you an example of our employee dedication. We had a night bellman who went with a guest to the hospital (the guest had appendicitis) and stayed all night there with him. That's who we are."

Employees, as Schulze taught, don't want to perform a function. Workers want to be part of a team and achieve a goal together. They want to be treated like a human being, and to act with humanity and warmth. Ritz Carlton employees are given leeway to serve customers directly to meet their needs, up to a $2000 budget. Giving workers the freedom to act independently on the customers' behalf makes the employee a stakeholder, a partner, and a pivotal team member, not just an employee.

Too many times in the modern working world, employees are treated like machines performing a function, or worse like helpless children, instead of important and capable people with dignity. Workers and customers are too often treated like numbers in a spreadsheet instead of *"ladies and gentlemen"* as they are at Ritz Carlton. Healthy work is about what's good, meaningful, and it's about creating the best in all of us, not just getting by.

The preceding case studies are idealistic but realistic cases of companies engaged in Healthy Work. Why not shoot for the moon? If Patagonia, Chick-fil-A, The Lodge Cast Iron Co, and Ritz-Carlton Hotels did it, why can't you? Why not create work that matters? Why not be bold, be courageous, and care? Why not give the best we can, to our employees, our employers, our customers, clients, and fellow citizens?

This is what *Healthy Work* is all about. Work is a good thing. It builds our culture and makes our lives better. Work, trade and commerce create wealth, peace, and happiness if done in a healthy way. These businesses did it and so can you.

8

Questions, Exercises, & Tips for Healthy Work

"The superior man seeks within; the inferior man seeks within others."
- *Confucius*

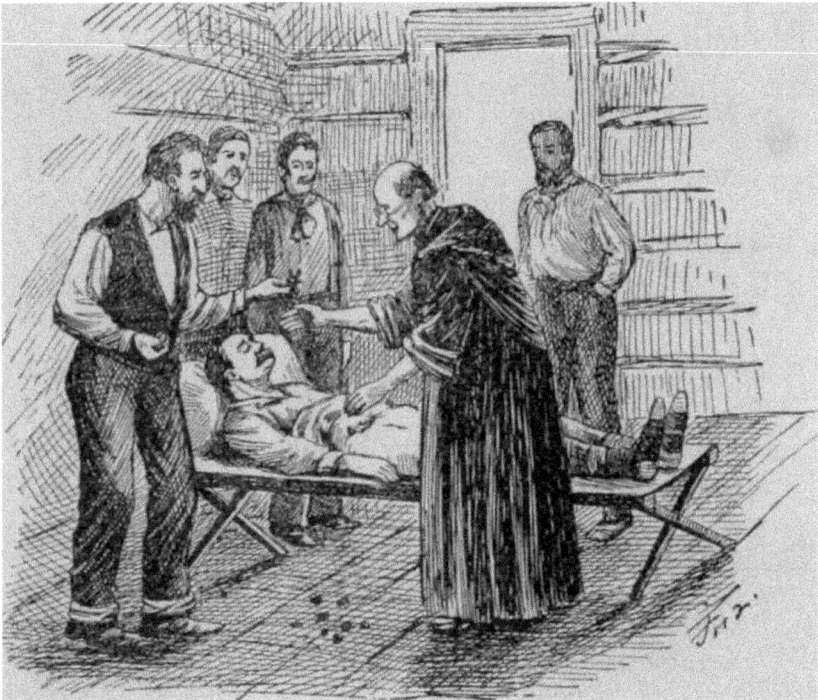

A Country Doctor, 1891

As we covered in a previous chapter, healthy work is both a _spiritual_ task- being connected to something lasting and transcendent, a _mental_ task- challenging ourselves to learn and grow in our career, and a _physical_ task- taking care of our physical health at work. Now that we know what healthy work is, let's use the following questions as prompts to explore and learn more about ourselves and our working lives. Use a journal to go through and answer each question. Then formulate a plan to implement what you learn. Keep it simple, but take action after you complete the exercises.

Spiritual Health at Work - The Big Picture

- What are you doing right now that is scary and hard?

- How are you contributing at work?

- What is the most important thing about your work?

- Who are you bringing together at work?

- What is scarce that you can uniquely provide?

- What are you good at?

- What fires you up?

- What would you like to change?

- What does a better world, city, neighborhood, place of work, family, and personal life look like to you?

Big Picture Tips:

- Have one unifying theme or value that controls the others, love, for example, and which will motivate you to work hard.

- Connect to institutions or create things yourself which leave behind a positive legacy when you're gone.

- Rule your inner world like a wise and just ruler would rule his kingdom.

- It's not about what you "feel like doing", it's about what needs to get done.

- *Values* should drive *goals*, which should drive *objectives* and *projects*.

Mental Health at Work

- What distracts you and how can you eliminate distractions?

- What are you doing at work which isn't important and that you could stop doing?

- Are you setting a few simple and achievable but challenging goals? What are they?

- Do you worry and obsess about things that don't matter?

- Are you harboring corrosive resentment, anger, lust, rage, or jealousy at work? What should you focus on instead? How can you resolve these issues?

Mental Tips

- Write out your values and then goals, then the objectives and projects required to reach each goal and live out each value.

- Learn to re-frame negative situations into a constructive context.

- Pray, meditate, or use a mantra or deep breathing exercises to take away negative and destructive emotions, stress, and worry.

- Establish personal growth daily rituals such as reading 30 minutes every morning, exercising 30 minutes, or briefly reviewing your goals daily.

- When you feel overwhelmed, break down overwhelm into pieces. Take a step back and view this problem from the bigger picture. Think small.

- Get outside a few minutes every day if possible to clear your head.

- Learn to re-calibrate and re-focus when your mind wanders, and you will not be captive to thoughts and emotions.

- Talk to someone about work, about your frustrations and ambitions, and learn to externalize what you're going through.

Physical Health at Work

- Are you active throughout the day?

- Are you sitting with good posture, and lifting with good posture throughout the day?

- Are you getting enough sunlight, at least 10-15 minutes per day?

- How often do you get up and move around at work?

- How much sugar, fried food, and processed carbohydrates do you eat?

- Do you take a break from your work every few hours?

- Can you find a quiet place to work?

Physical Tips

- Set out your exercise clothes the night before and you'll be more likely to do it.

- Exercise in the morning and you will do it more often. Plus, morning exercise boosts your mood and improves your focus, memory, and energy at work.

- Prepare healthy food and snacks before the week starts.

- Eat fruits, nuts, and vegetables as snacks.

- Fiber makes you feel full and less hungry, and helps you eat less.

- Intermittent fasting can be helpful for weight loss.

- Get down on the floor and stretch every day.

- Drink plenty of water.

- Lactic acid triggers chemicals in the brain which kill pain, so exercise is a powerful pain killer.

- Simplify.

- Motivation comes from a Latin root word which means "movement" so *move*, and you will be motivated.

9

Practical Principles of Healthy Work

& The Healthy Work Model™

1. Work should be celebrated as good in and of itself.

2. Work should be done to create value and fulfill human needs and desires.

3. Work should create value while doing no harm.

4. Work should be meaningful, constructive, and sustaining of human life to be healthy.

5. Work should uphold the right values.

6. Work should integrate and be healthy for the mind, body, and the spirit.

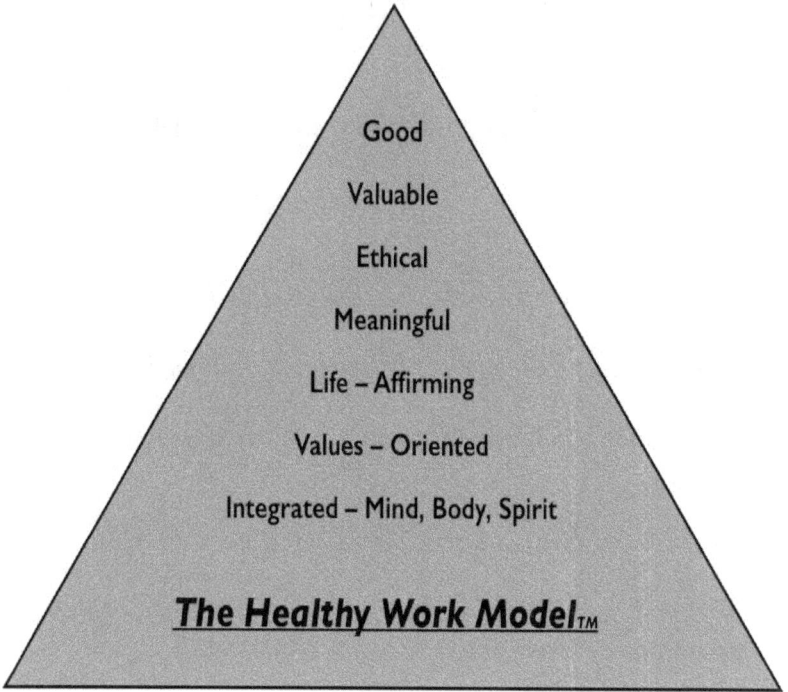

Good

Valuable

Ethical

Meaningful

Life – Affirming

Values – Oriented

Integrated – Mind, Body, Spirit

_The Healthy Work Model__{TM}

The End

Work is such a crucial part of life. It's not the only part, but it's important and worth taking some time to reflect on. Be proud of your work because work is a noble undertaking. Healthy work creates value, healthy work gives us a way to make a living, and healthy work can even be fun and rewarding. There is beauty in the way a newspaper column is written, a truck driven, a class taught, or a meal cooked and delivered to the table. All work has value. All healthy work matters. All work done right is something we should be proud of. Despite all the tumult, upheaval, and changes going on all around us in the world, healthy work is a way of life for many, and it can be for you too. Go make it happen.

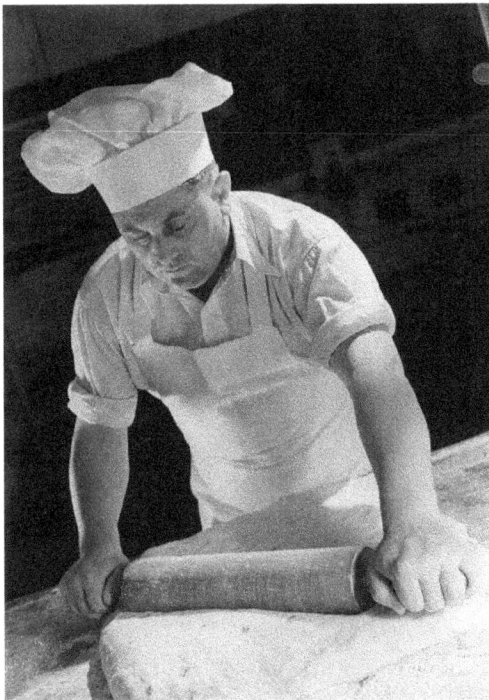

Baker, 1921

Cited Sources

1. Pew Research, 2015. www.pewresearch.com

2. McLean, Bethany, & Elkind, Peter. *The Smartest Guys in the Room: The Amazing Rise & Scandalous Fall of Enron.* Nov. 2013

3. *Volkswagen: The scandal explained.* Russell Hotten Business reporter. BBC News. Dec. 2015

4. Don Jacobs, Ashleigh Portales. Sexual Forensics: Lust, Passion, and Psychopathic Killers. 2014.

5. *Your Next Move.* Harvard Business Review. Summer 2015.

6. Godwin, Scott. *Movement & Meaning.* Roots Publishing August 2015.

7. Haidt, Jonathan. *The Righteous Mind.* February 2013.

8. Williams, Sam. CEO as Urban Statesman. December 2014.

9. Photos: Flickr, Creative Commons, No Known Copyright License

Other Sources & Suggested Reading

Small is Beautiful: Economics as if People Mattered by EF Schumacher

Understanding Michael Porter by Joan Magretta

Financial Markets Course, Yale University, Robert Shiller

The 7 Habits of Highly Effective People by Franklin Covey

Zen & the Art of Motorcycle Maintenance by Robert Pirsig

English Standard Version Bible

Human Action by Ludwig Von Mises

The Personal MBA by Josh Kaufman

Lynchpin by Seth Godin

The Brand Gap by Marty Neumeier

The Abolition of Man by CS Lewis

Sustainable Development Course, Dr. Jeffrey Sachs

The Ecology of Commerce by Paul Hawken

Brain Rules by John Medina

Max Weber's The Iron Cage of Bureaucracy

Aristotle's Nicomachean Ethics

The Righteous Mind by Jonathan Haidt

Bowling Alone by Charles Murray

Coming Apart by Charles Murray

Acedia: Metaphysical Boredom in the Empire of Desire by RJ Snell